Sandra Isabel Hernández González
Aurora Martínez-Romero
José Luis Ortega-Sánchez

Pharmacognosy Laboratory Manual

Sandra Isabel Hernández González
Aurora Martínez-Romero
José Luis Ortega-Sánchez

Pharmacognosy Laboratory Manual

Study of drugs and medicines of biological, plant, animal, microbiological origin and their derivatives.

ScienciaScripts

Cover image: www.ingimage.com

This book is a translation from the original published under ISBN 978-620-0-04491-4.

Publisher:
Sciencia Scripts
is a trademark of
Dodo Books Indian Ocean Ltd. and OmniScriptum S.R.L publishing group

120 High Road, East Finchley, London, N2 9ED, United Kingdom
Str. Armeneasca 28/1, office 1, Chisinau MD-2012, Republic of Moldova, Europe
Printed at: see last page
ISBN: 978-620-7-06231-7

LABORATORY MANUAL

PHARMACOGNOSY

Academic Body

In Consolidation

Diagnostic Medical Bacteriology and Public Health

UJED-CA-125

Dr. Sandra Isabel Hernández González
Dr. Aurora Martínez Romero
Dr. José Luis Ortega Sánchez
Dr. José de Jesús Alba Romero

2019

Prologue

The word pharmacognosy comes from the Greek *pharmakon* = remedy, drug. gnosis = *knowledge* "Knowledge of drugs", a term first used by Seydler in Analecta Pharmacognostica (1815). Pharmacognosy is considered a branch of pharmacology, the science that deals with the study of drugs and medicinal substances of natural, vegetable, microbial and animal origin.

It is the pharmacological science that deals with the knowledge of the raw material of biological origin that the pharmacist or the pharmaceutical industry uses for the preparation of drugs under certain pharmaceutical forms. It has evolved along with human thought, responding to vital survival needs. It is the embryonic science of pharmacological sciences, of the rudiments of medicine.

It requires knowledge of botany, biology, pharmacodynamics, pharmacology, galenic pharmacy, pharmacokinetics, pharmaceutical technology, toxicology, plant and animal physiology, biochemistry and organic chemistry, mainly; in some way, all disciplines contribute to the knowledge of the effect of natural or synthetic active ingredients on living organisms.

The purpose of this pharmacognosy practice manual is to introduce the student to the study and application of pharmacognosy. Its content is theoretical and written in such a way as to facilitate its comprehension. It presents 16 practices to be performed without the need of sophisticated equipment, only with the material to perform routine conventional tests, under the principle of always working with responsibility, commitment and professional ethics. As criteria for the selection of the practices, the need for the Pharmaceutical Chemist Biologist student to acquire solid training, ability and competence necessary to solve problems in the area of pharmacognosy with the basic knowledge of quality and application of natural products in the development of new products was visualized as the criteria for the selection of the practices.

TABLE OF CONTENTS

Introduction

The word pharmacognosy comes from the Greek *pharmakon* = drug, gnosis = knowledge. Pharmacognosy can be defined as the branch of pharmaceutical sciences that studies drugs and medicines of biological origin, be it vegetable, animal or microbiological, and their derivatives. This includes what are known as natural products, mainly of medicinal interest, but not limited only to such substances.

Traditionally in Pharmacy, studies on products and materials used as drugs were called "Materia Medica".

In 1817 the German pharmacist was the one who introduced the term Pharmacognosy. It should be borne in mind that at the beginning of the 19th century, chemistry did not exist as an independent science and that as chemical theories and knowledge advanced, both areas became inextricably linked.

Many of these common subjects are known as "Phytochemistry", "Natural Products" or "Herbalism" among chemically oriented scientific subjects. At present, these terms may not be very satisfactory given the great progress in all branches of the science of Chemistry and Pharmacy, in which "active ingredient", "semi-synthetic drugs", "synthetic drugs" already appear.

In a broad sense, Pharmacognosy encompasses knowledge of the history, trade, distribution and geography, botany, cultivation, collection, selection, preparation and preservation, identification and evaluation by all types of methods, chemical composition and traditional use of drugs and their derivatives to improve the health of man or other animals. All types of plant drugs and other natural products that have commercial value for their technological uses, including a variety of products for commercial use, among them colorants, flavorings, condiments, insecticides, herbicides, antibiotics, allergenic extracts, and biological immunizers, etc.

History of pharmacognosy and its importance today

The use of plants to treat diseases and ailments is one of the characteristics of human beings since their appearance on earth. Remains of medicinal plants that are still used today have been found in excavations made in places inhabited prehistorically by man. It is also known that some animals, including primates, used and continue to use plants to combat certain diseases such as parasitic diseases. Perhaps the use of plants was initiated by man by imitation with certain animals, to later become a study that to date continues as "popular" wisdom, which is still transmitted orally.

In his long struggle against the blind forces of nature, man found in plants an ally, they provided him with a roof, shelter, weapons, a remedy for pain and even solace for the spirit. The great amount of energy that the plant has to grow, to develop and to be reborn every season made that the peoples, from the most primitive to the advanced ones have attributed magical powers to certain species and that so many myths and legends have arisen that confer to them a direct intervention in the life of the man and in his destiny.

In all ancient civilizations such as Greece, Persia, Egypt, Rome, etc., and we know the importance that the ancient Mexicans gave to the knowledge about plants and their attributes, which was reflected in their daily existence, thanks to Don Francisco Hernandez (1517-1587) Spanish physician, botanist and archaeologist, he was the chamber physician of Philip II. In 1570 and 1577 he directed the scientific expedition that herborized the flora of New Spain and in which he revalued the indigenous botanical and therapeutic knowledge, his work is found under the title of *"Rerum medicarum novae Hispaniae thesaurus" (*1628), in the part dedicated to the botanical gardens of Anahuac, as the love for plants and flowers was given from the lowest social strata, to the Mexican nobility itself. Nezahualcoyotl king acolhua, was the founder of the first botanical gardens located in Tetzcotzinco, Quauhyacae and Tzinacanoztoc. Likewise, the iconography of the Mexica played an important role in the description of the plants by those in charge of drawing the plants for their later recognition "tlahcuilos". This same historian maintains that the Nahua had a systematic classification similar in some ways to that of Linnaeus.

Nowadays, there is more virtual information, written, either in books, magazines, etc., through which the dissemination of the study and research on plants is easily accessible to the student without neglecting the history of herbal medicine throughout our territory.

The laboratory practices in the teaching of Pharmacognosy have a very important role in the learning process in the elaboration of pharmaceuticals, within the practice it is sought that the student works in compliance with the rules of hygiene, responsibility and professional ethics as well as to put into practice their skills, abilities, and use their ingenuity in the marketing of the products produced, so that in the future it may be the area of career exploitation.

Mission of the QFB program

It is a quality educational program oriented to the integral formation of professionals in the area of Chemical, Pharmaceutical and Biological Sciences, free, responsible and competitive with humanistic and ethical values that generate and apply knowledge in the pharmaceutical, environmental preservation and biomedical sectors, linking them in a timely manner and with a bioethical sense with the productive, social and scientific sectors, contributing to the progress of the State and the Country.

Vision of the QFB program

By 2020, the Biological Pharmaceutical Chemist educational program of the School of Chemical Sciences in Gomez Palacio will have the corresponding Accreditation, with consolidated academic bodies that favor the formation of certified professionals, with great research capacity and high spirit of service, supported by a broad linkage with all social actors to contribute to the social, economic and scientific development of the country.

Table of competencies

Compete nce to Acquire	Target	Context	Rank or status	Performance criteria	Scientific Basis
The student knows how to apply the knowledge of Pharmacognosy in professional practice and possesses the intellectual skills necessary for such practice.	Analyze and reason the relationship between theory and practice.	Laboratory processing of pharmaceuticals with pyrogen- and toxin-free material	They will serve as a basis for the production of various medicines.	Acquisition of skills and abilities that allow him/her to know about the type of laboratory instruments and materials for the elaboration of pharmaceutical dosage forms.	Knowledge of the different techniques for the elaboration of different medicines.

Performance Level

The set of practices in this manual will allow you to reach a level 4 performance according to the CONOCER classification, namely, in Level 4 you develop a set of activities of diverse nature, in which you have to show creativity and resources to reconcile interests. They must have the ability to motivate and lead work groups.

The reasons we assume you will achieve a high level of performance are:

1. The completion of the internship in a timely manner presupposes the mastery of different skills and knowledge.
2. The preparation of a protocol and a practice report requires discipline and hard work, as well as the use of computational tools.
3. The internships must be done individually, since each student will produce their drugs throughout the semester working under the name of a laboratory that will be responsible for manufacturing and commercialization.

The number of students per group to be worked with is a maximum of 25, the practice for the importance it has in the career will be individually, for which each student will work as responsible for a laboratory, which will have the name of their choice, each one will be responsible for the preparation, packaging, packaging, labeling of each of the products that are produced throughout the course, this is intended to raise awareness of the student of the responsibility and professional ethics of their work.

The evaluation will be made according to the presentation of the finished product, which must meet the requirements set by the quality standards, which the teacher will be responsible for giving the relevant indications in case the labeling or packaging is not well for its return, until it completes the requirement. The student will present along with the product for its revision, a monograph of each one of the ingredients that enter in the elaboration of the product also for its revision, as part of the evaluation.

Evaluation system

Performance evaluation

1. You must submit your report by the deadline set by the teacher and include the following items:

a. Deliver the finished product, duly packaged and labeled according to the regulations of the general health law on advertising (official journal of the federation of May 4, 2000) in articles 42 and 43 and the Mexican Official Standard.

b. Submit the internship report which should include the following:

1. Cover page with the name of the laboratory you selected, with the data requested according to pharmacy labeling standards. Place the laboratory's own logo and the data requested by the Secretary of Health for Pharmaceutical Responsiva.

2. On the second sheet: the formula of the drug, including dosage and precautions and contraindications for its use.

3. In the following pages you will find the monographs of all the ingredients that are part of the formula, including the formula and chemical structure of the ingredients, and bibliography consulted.

Note: Submitting the report does not indicate that the practice has been completed for satisfactory evaluation, in case there are errors in the product these will be returned for correction and only then it can be evaluated.

Appraisal assignment

Attendance, punctuality	20%
2. Knowledge of practice and performance in the laboratory.	30 %
3. Delivery of the product correctly packaged and labeled.	25%
4. Delivery of corrected final report	25 %

General Safety Practices

The different regulations related to laboratory work in general are taken into account, such as:

Miscellaneous Regulations:

- General Law of Global Ecological Equilibrium
- General Health Law 11-VI-2009
- Federal Regulations on Safety, Hygiene and the Working Environment 21-I-1997

UJED Regulations:

- Organic Law of the UJED
- UJED General Regulations

FCQ Regulations

- FCQ Internal Regulations
- FCQ Laboratory Regulations
- Biochemistry Laboratory Regulations
- Biosafety Manual for the Pharmacy Laboratory

Mexican Official Standard

NOM-001-SPTS-2008	Buildings, premises, facilities and areas in the workplace - Safety conditions
NOM.002.STPS-2000	Safety, prevention, protection and firefighting conditions in the workplace.
NOM-005-STPS-1998	Related to safety and hygiene conditions in workplaces for the handling, transport and storage of hazardous chemical substances.
NOM-018-STPS-2000	System for the Identification and Communication of Hazards and Risks from Chemical Substances in the Work Centers-System
NOM-026-STPS-2008	Safety and hygiene colors and signs, and identification of risks due to fluids conducted in pipelines.
NOM-114-STPS-1996	System for the communication and identification of risks due to chemical substances in the Chemical Centers. Job
NOM-087-ECOL-SSA1-2002	Environmental protection - Environmental health - Biological and infectious hazardous waste - Classification and handling specifications.
NOM-052-SEMARNAT-2005	Which establishes the characteristics, identification procedure, classification and lists of hazardous wastes.
NOM-054-SEMARNAT-1993	Establishing the procedure to determine the incompatibility between two or more wastes considered as hazardous by NOM- 052- SEMARNAT-1993.
NOM-072-SSA1-1993	Drug Labeling April 10, 2000

Pharmacognosy Laboratory. Biosafety Manual

Introduction

Safety measures in laboratories are a set of preventive measures designed to protect the health of those who work there against the risks arising from the activity, to avoid accidents and contamination both within their work environment, as well as to the outside. The basic rules indicated here are a set of common sense practices carried out routinely.

The key element is the proactive attitude towards safety and the information that allows to recognize and combat the risks present in the laboratory. The meticulous performance of each technique will be fundamental, since no measure, not even excellent equipment, can replace the order and care with which one must work.

Target

The teaching and research activities carried out in the Pharmacognosy Laboratory of the School of Chemical Sciences of the Universidad Juárez del Estado de Durango involve risks when investigating new active ingredients that may constitute a starting point for the design of new drugs in the future, providing the student with basic knowledge about natural products, their quality requirements and application in pharmacognosy, always under the control of biosafety measures.

Regulation

Order is essential to avoid accidents

1. You must enter the laboratory with white coat, long sleeves, preferably cotton, closed shoes, avoiding the use of hanging accessories on the neck or long earrings that endanger the safety of the practitioner.
2. Know the location of safety elements in the workplace, such as: fire extinguishers, emergency exits, fire blankets, eye wash, spill containment tray,

alarms, etc.

3. Reagent bottles and some devices may display icons and phrases informing about their dangerousness, correct use and measures to be taken in case of ingestion, inhalation, etc. Read this information carefully and take into account the specifications indicated therein.

4. Eating, drinking, smoking or wearing make-up is prohibited.

5. It is forbidden to store food in the laboratory or in the laboratory refrigerators.

6. It is essential to maintain order and cleanliness. Each person is directly responsible for his or her assigned area and all common areas.

7. Hands should be washed thoroughly before and after any laboratory handling and before leaving the laboratory.

8. Appropriate gloves should be worn to avoid contact with toxic chemicals or infectious biological material. Any person whose gloves are contaminated should not touch objects or surfaces, such as: telephone, pencils, drawer or door handles, notebooks, etc.

9. Mouth pipetting will not be allowed.

10. Pay attention to the name of the dilutions and products before using them.

11. Keep the work area tidy, free of books, coats, bags, excess chemical bottles and unnecessary or useless things.

12. Work should be unhurried, thinking at all times about what is being done, and with the material and reagents in order.

13. Never force a glass tube, since, in case of breakage, the cuts can be serious.

14. The hot glass should be set aside on an iron or similar until it cools. If in doubt, use tongs or pliers.

15. Never use glass equipment that is cracked or broken. Dispose of broken glassware in a glass container, not in the traditional trash can.

16. If an intense heat source is used, move chemical reagent bottles away from the source.

17. Never heat flammable liquids with a lighter.

18. A possible poisoning hazard, often overlooked, is through the skin. Avoid skin

contact with chemicals, especially those that are toxic or corrosive (acids and alkalis), by wearing disposable gloves.

19. Wash hands often

20. Reagent bottles are always transported by the bottom, never by the stopper.

21. Do not drop containers or displace hot liquid.

22. Never heat a completely closed container.

23. Always point the mouth of the container away from yourself and others nearby.

24. No horseplay, running, playing, pushing, etc. in the laboratory.

25. Each team must be in charge of collecting the material, eliminating waste and leaving their lab table perfectly tidy, following the teacher's instructions.

26. Whenever necessary protect eyes and face from splashes or impacts. Safety glasses, visors or face shields or other protective devices should be used when handling chemicals that emit vapors or may cause splashing.

27. To avoid accidental electric shock, follow the operating and handling instructions of the equipment exactly.

28. Avoid handling liquids in the proximity of electrical instruments and be careful with thermostatized baths.

29. Never plug in equipment with cables or connections in poor condition.

30. Never handle inside an appliance, even when disconnected from the power supply.

31. Do not wear contact lenses in the laboratory, since, in the event of an accident, chemical splashes or their vapors may pass behind the lenses and cause eye injuries.

32. Do not inhale, taste or smell chemicals if you are not properly informed.

33. Never bring the nose close to inhale directly from a test tube or container with liquid.

34. Emergency exits or aisles should not be blocked with equipment, machines or other elements that hinder proper circulation.

35. Any corrosive, toxic, flammable, oxidizing, radioactive, explosive or noxious material must be properly labeled.

36. The use of disposable masks is required when there is a risk of producing aerosols (mixture of particles in a liquid medium) or dusts during weighing operations of toxic substances.

37. Practices that produce gases, vapors, fumes or particles, those that may be hazardous by inhalation must be carried out under a hood.

38. The absence of flammable vapors should be verified before igniting an ignition source. Do not operate flammable materials or solvents on or near direct flame.

39. Broken glass material should not be deposited with common waste. It should be placed in sturdy boxes, wrapped in paper and inside plastic bags.

40. Any container that has contained flammable material and must be discarded must be completely emptied, drained, rinsed with an appropriate solvent and then rinsed with water several times.

41. It is prohibited to discharge flammable or toxic or corrosive liquids or biological material down the drains of sinks, toilets or common waste containers. In each case, the established procedures for waste management must be followed. Consult with the teacher or with the people in charge of the laboratory.

42. When storing chemical substances, consider that there are a certain number of them that are incompatible because when stored together they can give rise to dangerous reactions. Before storing chemicals, consult the safety manual of the Multidisciplinary Laboratory of the Faculty of Chemical Sciences in Gómez Palacio.

43. The laboratories will have a first aid kit with the essential elements to attend emergency cases.

44. The person in charge of the Laboratory, or the Laboratory Technicians, will be informed when it is necessary to leave the equipment working in the absence of the person in charge of the practice.

45. It is not allowed to perform any activity in the laboratory if it is not authorized by the teacher.

Emergency procedures

Medical emergencies

If an emergency occurs such as: injuries, burns, accidental ingestion of a chemical, toxic or dangerous product, fainting or fainting, you should proceed:

1. The injured will be provided with first aid.
2. Simultaneously, the Head of Laboratory will be notified.
3. The Head of Laboratory will notify the Direction of the Faculty of Chemical Sciences of the accident,

Fire:

1. Stay calm. The most important thing is to get to safety and warn others.
2. If there is an alarm, sound it. If not, shout to alert others.
3. Immediate notice shall be given to the management offices, informing the place and characteristics of the loss, so that they may take the pertinent measures.
4. If the fire is small and you know how to use an extinguisher, use it. If the fire is serious, do not take any risks and keep calm and implement the evacuation plan.
5. If you must evacuate the area, turn off electrical equipment and close gas valves and windows.
6. Evacuate the area by the assigned route.
7. Do not run, walk fast, closing as many doors as possible. Do not use elevators. Descend whenever possible.
8. Do not carry objects with you, they may hinder your exit.
9. If you were unable to exit for any reason, please re-enter. Let the specialized teams take care of it.

Chemical spill

1. Attend to anyone who may have been affected.
2. Notify people in nearby areas near the spill. Place demarcation tape to warn of the hazard.
3. Evacuate all non-essential persons from the spill area.

4. If the spill is of flammable material, extinguish sources of ignition, and heat sources.
5. Avoid breathing vapors of spilled material, if necessary use a respiratory mask with filters appropriate to the type of spill.
6. Ventilate the area.
7. Use personal protective equipment such as clothing resistant to acids, bases and organic solvents and gloves.
8. Confine or contain the spill, preventing it from spreading. To do this, extend the cords around the spill.
9. Then absorb the spill with appropriate utensils.
10. Leave to act and then shovel up and place the residue in the red bag and seal it.
11. If the spill is of a highly volatile element, leave the bag with the waste inside the hood until it is removed for disposal.
12. Wash spill area with soap and water. Dry thoroughly.
13. Carefully remove and clean up all items that may have been splashed by the spill.
14. Wash gloves, mask and clothing.

FLOWCHART OF THE PROCEDURE TO IDENTIFY THE HAZARDOUSNESS OF A WASTE (LISTING AND CHARACTERIZATION)

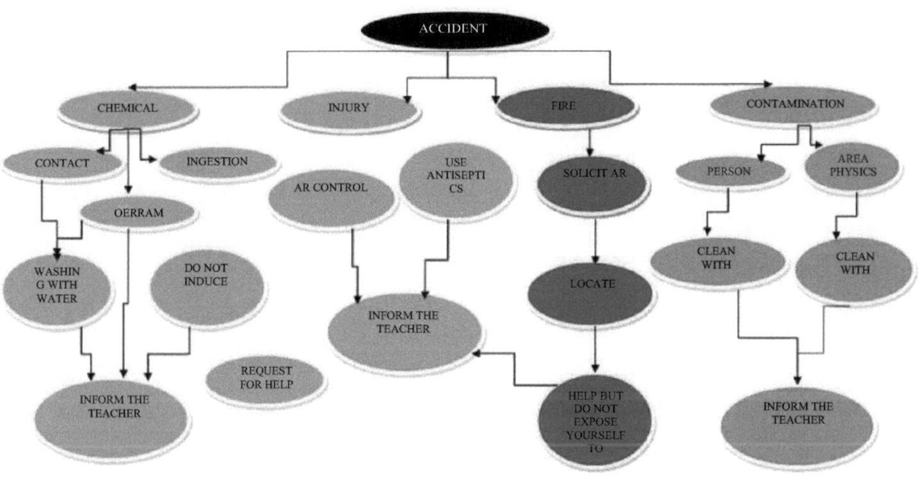

Practice 1. Effervescent Powders

Introduction

Powders are one of the oldest dosage forms in existence. However, nowadays most pharmaceutical products appear in forms other than powders, such as tablets and capsules.

The first formulations of these effervescent powders date back to 1824 and are attributed to Tomas Savory, who named them Seidlitz powders (a spring in Germany which had the therapeutic properties of magnesium sulfate).

Target

Elaborate the effervescent powders to know the role played by each of the ingredients of the formula provided by the teacher, determining the compatibility or incompatibility of each one of them, for possible modification if necessary, without altering the therapeutic action. Once the drug is finished, proceed to the primary and secondary packaging and labeling of the drug according to the established norms.

Basis

Effervescent powders are a presentation for oral administration in the form of unidosis containing acidic substances and bicarbonates that react rapidly in water releasing CO2. They are intended for dissolution or dispersion in water prior to administration.

Formula:

Sodium Bicarbonate	2.5 g
Tartaric Acid	0.200 g
Citric Acid	2.0 g
Starchq.s.	5.0 g

- These quantities are for one dose. They will be wrapped in paper. Make for 10 doses.
- Papers or ballots: These are distributions of powders in equal doses that are wrapped in flattened paper packages, as if they were envelopes.
- The paper has to be rectangular and of satin surface. The totality of the powders is prepared and divided in "n" parts in the "n" prepared papers.
- Once the powder has been distributed, the weighing should be checked individually.

Material

1. Mortar
2. Spatula
3. Granatary balance
4. Disposable surgical gloves

All the material must be perfectly clean, preferably washed with: water, soap, rinsed with potable water, distilled water, alcohol and dried.

Experimental part

1. Mix the reagents in a mortar and pestle, and distribute on the wrapping papers.
2. The teacher will always be present during the practice to solve any problems that may arise.
3. Once the papers are prepared, they are labeled, and the ten doses requested are placed in a secondary container and labeled according to Mexican packaging and labeling standards.
4. The labeling of the product shall be carried out as indicated in the theoretical class and is in accordance with the standards.

Practice 2. Acetylsalicylic acid capsules

Introduction

Gelatin capsules are preparations of solid consistency formed by a hard or soft shell of variable shape and capacity, usually containing a single dose of medication. They are almost always intended for oral administration. The shell is usually gelatin and its consistency (hard or soft) is achieved by the addition of substances such as glycerol and sorbitol. Each capsule is made up of 2 parts, the larger part which is the receptacle in which the drug is placed and the smaller part which acts as a cap.

Target

Identify the parts and consistency of the capsules, as well as fill them with the established ingredient.

Basis

The elaboration of acetylsalicylic acid capsules for oral administration is one of those favored by pharmaceutical marketing to facilitate the release of the drug in the stomach. The capsules to be chosen will be those with the capacity indicated in the formula.

Formula:

Acetylsalicylic acid 500 mg

Material

1. Granatary balance
2. Spatula. Make 10 capsules with the same dose each.

Experimental part

1. To fill the capsules, the capsules are manually uncapped, the receptacles are placed in rows on paper as close together as possible; the powder placed on glossy paper is divided equally. The lids are placed one at a time on the receptacles, pressing gently and turning at the same time. The surface is cleaned with a soft cloth.
2. The teacher will always be present for any problems or doubts that may arise.
3. Once the capsules have been prepared, primary and secondary packaging and labeling are carried out in accordance with Mexican labeling and packaging standards.

Practice 3. Mentholated petroleum jelly

Introduction

The use of petroleum jelly as a vehicle for different drugs and active ingredients of medicinal plants is very old and the most economical is known as "simple ointment" when added to yellow wax.

Target

Identify each of the components and their association to evaluate possible side effects, as well as the role of the base (vaseline) as an excipient. The alcoholic extracts used in the practice are those previously prepared in Pharmacognosy I in the previous semester.

Basis

Vaseline also called petrolatum is a compound derived from petroleum which is used in pharmacy as an excipient of ointments, but it is not easily absorbed as other oily bases. Various associations of decongestants, antitussives, bronchodilators and expectorants can be used, especially with vegetable extracts.

Formula:

Solid Vaseline	100.0 g
Menthol (10% alcoholic solution)	10.0 mL
Camphor (5% alcoholic solution)	5.0 mL
Eucalyptus (alcoholic extract)	5.0 mL
Guaiacol (1% alcoholic solution)	3.0 mL

Material

1. Granatary balance
2. Metal spatula
3. 400 mL beaker
4. Bain Marie
5. Graduated pipettes for each of the 10 mL liquid ingredients

Experimental part

1. Melt the petroleum jelly in a Bain Marie (80°C).
2. Once melted, remove it from the bath and add (removed from any flame) the liquid ingredients mixing with the spatula until the alcohol evaporates. And the consistency of the ointment is homogeneous.
3. The teacher will always be present for any problems or doubts that may arise.
4. When the product has reached ambient temperature, proceed to primary and secondary packaging and labeling.

Practice 4. Antifungal ointment

Introduction

Semi-solid topical preparations are intended to be applied on the skin or on certain mucous membranes, with the purpose of exerting a local action, to carry out percutaneous penetration of active ingredients or for their emollient or protective action. Eudermic skin is the normal and ideal skin type, balanced in terms of hydration and natural oiliness that it should have, oil-in-water type. It has a light layer of grease that does not give an oily sheen to the surface. It does not present desquamation and it is very difficult to present pimples or impurities, it is the skin of babies and children. Ectodermal skin is the skin can be poorly pigmented, thin, although on palms and soles it can be thick and excessively fragile, prone to eczema, scratches, blisters and infections.

Target

Identify each of the components and their association to evaluate the possible side effects, as well as the role of the base (petroleum jelly) as an excipient. In the preparation of this product, mentholated petroleum jelly as prepared in the previous practice can be used as the base of the ointment.

Basis

Dermatological preparations can be classified into three groups, depending on the site of action of the active ingredients they contain:

1. Preparations with superficial action (eudermic preparations).
2. Preparations with dermal action (ectodermal preparations).
3. Preparations with systemic action.

The preparation to be prepared is No. 1 because in this classification the ointment must remain on the surface of the skin, in the place where they have been applied. They are used for the treatment of certain conditions of the epidermis. An example of this type are antibiotic ointments.

Formula:

Solid petroleum jelly or mentholated petroleum jelly	50 g
Yellow arnica (alcoholic extract)	2.0 mL
Thyme (alcoholic extract)	2.0 mL
Cancer herb	2.0 mL
Grass in Cross	2.0 mL
Parsley (alcoholic extract)	2.0 mL
Acetic acid	1.0 mL
Sassafras Oil	0.5 mL
5% Iodide Iodide Solution	1.0 mL
Sulfur	0.5 g

Material

1. 400 mL glass beaker
2. Metal spatula
3. Granatary balance
4. Graduated glass pipettes for% each extract, 5 ml each

Experimental part

1. Melt the petroleum jelly in a Bain Marie (80°C).
2. Once melted, remove it from the bath and add (removed from any flame) the liquid ingredients mixing with the spatula until the alcohol evaporates.
3. The sulfur should be mixed separately with a small portion of the same petroleum jelly before mixing it with the rest of the formulation because lumps may form that are difficult to break up.
4. Continue mixing until a homogeneous consistency is obtained.
5. The teacher will always be present for any problems or doubts that may arise.
6. When the product has reached ambient temperature, proceed to primary and secondary packaging and labeling.

Practice 5. Analgesic Ointment I

Introduction

The use of petroleum jelly as a vehicle for different drugs and active ingredients of medicinal plants is very old and the most economical, and known when it is added with yellow wax it is known as "simple ointment". However, it can be prepared with petroleum jelly alone and is considered a hydrophobic ointment.

Target

Identify each of the components and their association to evaluate possible side effects, as well as the role of the base (petroleum jelly) as excipient.

Basis

Analgesic ointments are preparations of soft consistency containing the active material(s) and additives incorporated into an appropriate base that gives it mass and consistency. This base can be liposoluble or hydrosoluble, generally anhydrous or with a maximum of 20% water. When it contains a washable or water removable base, it is also called hydrophilic ointment. The routes of administration are topical.

Formula:

Solid petroleum jelly	100 g
Yellow arnica (alcoholic extract)	5.0 mL
Camphor	5.0 g
Cane alcohol	5.0 mL

Material

1. 400 mL glass beaker
2. Metal spatula
3. Granatary balance
4. 5 mL graduated glass pipette
5. Test tube with sufficient capacity to dissolve the camphor in the 5 mL of alcohol
6. The teacher will always be present for any problems or doubts that may arise.

Experimental part

1. Melt the petroleum jelly in a water bath (80°C).
2. Remove it from the water bath (and removed from any flame) and when it is at room temperature add the camphor solution and arnica extract, mixing constantly until the alcohol evaporates and the mixture is homogeneous.
3. Proceed to primary and secondary packaging and labeling of the product.

Practice 6. Analgesic Ointment II

Introduction

The use of petroleum jelly as a vehicle for different drugs and active ingredients of medicinal plants is very old and the most economical, and known when added to yellow wax is known as "simple ointment". However, it can be prepared with petroleum jelly alone and is considered a hydrophobic ointment.

Target

Identify each of the components and their association to evaluate possible side effects, as well as the role of the base (petroleum jelly) as excipient.

Basis

Analgesic ointments are preparations of soft consistency containing the active material(s) and additives incorporated into an appropriate base that gives it mass and consistency. This base can be liposoluble or hydrosoluble, generally anhydrous or with a maximum of 20% water. When it contains a washable or water removable base, it is also called hydrophilic ointment. The routes of administration are topical

Formula:

Liquid petroleum jelly	50.0mL
Solid petroleum jelly	50.0 mL
3. Methyl salicylate (10% alcoholic solution)	2.0 mL

Liquid petroleum jelly 50.0mL

4. 5% iodized solution 2.0 mL

Material

1. 400 mL glass beaker
2. Granatary balance
3. 5 mL glass pipettes one for each solution used
4. Glass stirrer
5. Bain Marie

Experimental part

1. Melt the petroleum jelly in a water bath (80°C).
2. Remove it from the water bath (and removed from any flame) and when it is at room temperature add the rest of the ingredients, stirring constantly until the alcohol evaporates and the mixture is homogeneous.
3. Proceed to primary and secondary packaging and labeling of the product.
4. The teacher will always be present for any problems or doubts that may arise.

Practice 7. Analgesic Ointment III

Introduction

The use of petroleum jelly as a vehicle for different drugs and active ingredients of medicinal plants is very old and the most economical, and known when it is added with yellow wax it is known as "simple ointment". However, it can be prepared with petroleum jelly alone and is considered a hydrophobic ointment.

Target

Identify each of the components and their association to evaluate possible side effects, as well as the role of the base (petroleum jelly) as excipient.

Basis

Analgesic ointments are preparations of soft consistency containing the active material(s) and additives incorporated into an appropriate base that gives it mass and consistency. This base can be liposoluble or water-soluble, generally anhydrous or with a maximum of 20% water. When it contains a washable or water removable base, it is also called hydrophilic ointment. The routes of administration are topical

Formula:

1. Solid petroleum jelly	100 g
2. Yellow arnica (alcoholic extract)	5.0 mL
3. Calendula (5% alcoholic solution)	5.0 mL
4.- Camphor (5 % alcoholic solution)	3.0 mL

Material

1. 400 mL glass beaker
2. Granatary balance
3. 5 mL glass pipettes one for each solution used
4. Glass stirrer
5. Bain Marie

Experimental part

1. Melt the petroleum jelly in a water bath (80°C).
2. Remove it from the water bath (and removed from any flame) and when it is at room temperature add the rest of the ingredients, stirring constantly until the alcohol evaporates and the mixture is homogeneous.
3. Proceed to primary and secondary packaging and labeling of the product.
4. The teacher will always be present for any problems or doubts that may arise.

Practice 8. Analgesic Ointment IV

Introduction

In medicine, an ointment or ointment is a galenic form composed of fats or similar substances, for the application of active ingredients to the skin. Ointments differ fundamentally from creams by the absence of water in their composition. Vaseline is a petroleum derivative, a mixture of aromatic hydrocarbons, with many beneficial qualities and uses, such as moisturizing the skin and lips. It is currently used in cosmetology and in the pharmaceutical industry.

The use of petroleum jelly as a vehicle for different drugs and active ingredients of medicinal plants is very old and the most economical, and known when added to yellow wax is known as "simple ointment". However, it can be prepared with petroleum jelly alone and is considered a hydrophobic ointment.

Target

Identify each of the components and their association to evaluate possible side effects, as well as the role of the base (petroleum jelly) as excipient.

Basis

Analgesic ointments are preparations of soft consistency containing the active material(s) and additives incorporated into an appropriate base that gives it mass and consistency. This base can be liposoluble or water-soluble, generally anhydrous or with a maximum of 20% water. When it contains a washable or water removable base, it is also called hydrophilic ointment. The routes of administration are topical.

Formula:

1. Solid petroleum jelly	100 g
2. Camphor	5.0 g
3. Cane alcohol (c.b.p. to dissolve camphor).	5.0 mL

Material

1. 400 mL glass beaker
2. Granatary balance
3. Metal spatula
4. 10 mL pipette
5. Bain Marie

Experimental part

1. Melt the petroleum jelly in a water bath (80°C).
2. Remove it from the water bath (and removed from any flame) and when it is at room temperature add the rest of the ingredients, stirring constantly until the alcohol evaporates and the mixture is homogeneous.
3. Proceed to primary and secondary packaging and labeling of the product.
4. The teacher will always be present for any problems or doubts that may arise.

Practice 9. Camphorated Oil

Introduction

In pharmacology, liniment is the name given to a preparation less thick than an ointment in which oils and balsams are used as a base and which is applied externally in frictions. At the beginning of the 20th century, a distinction was made between ammoniacal or volatile liniment, which is a mixture of liquid ammonia and olive or sweet almond oil that acts as an irritant, and calcareous liniment or oil, which is a mixture of equal parts of lime water and sweet almond or linseed oil. Liniments are another way of making topically applied drugs that are applied by rubbing (rubbing on the skin) on the affected area with an oily consistency, and that is why they were called" embrocations." They should not be applied to bruised or excoriated areas.

Target

Identify each of the components and their association to evaluate possible side effects, as well as the role of the base (vegetable oil, liquid petroleum jelly, glycerol, etc.) as excipient.

Basis

They are solutions or mixtures of various substances in oil, alcoholic solutions of soap or emulsions. They are intended for external application. The excipient (oil) must be of good quality, free of foreign matter and microorganisms.

Formula:

Vegetable oil	100 mL
2. Camphor	10.0 g
3. Cane alcohol (c.b.p. dissolve camphor)	5.0 mL

Material

1. Granatary balance
2. 250 mL glass beaker
3. 100 mL graduated cylinder
4. Granatary balance
5. Metal spatula
6. 10.0 mL glass pipette

Experimental part

1. Dissolve the camphor in the glass beaker with the cane alcohol, adding it 2 mL at a time and so on, until it is completely dissolved, shaking the beaker gently to aid dissolution.
2. The teacher will always be present for any problems or doubts that may arise.

Practice 10. Camphor Alcohol

Introduction

Another way of elaborating topical application drugs are liniments that are applied by rubbing the affected area with an alcoholic consistency, and that is why they were called "embrocations". They should not be applied on bruised or excoriated areas.

Target

Identify each of the components and their association to evaluate possible side effects, as well as the role of the base (alcohol, glycerol, etc.) as excipient.

Basis

They are usually preparations in alcohol or in alcohol and water are also often called liniments, like the oily ones are used for rubbing on the skin producing a cooling sensation, acts as a mild anesthetic, and for symptoms of fatigue.

Formula:

1. Cane alcohol	100 mL
2. Camphor	10 g

Material

1. 250 mL glass beaker
2. Granatary balance
3. Metal spatula
4. 100 mL flask

Experimental part

1. After measuring the alcohol add it to the camphor that will be in the glass, mix the glass gently until complete dissolution.
2. The teacher will always be present for any problems or doubts that may arise.

Practical 11. Fungicide Solution For Faneras (Nails)

Introduction

Fangs are complementary and visible structures on or protruding from the skin. Fangs are nails and hairs in humans and feathers, hooves, scales and horns in animals. Fangs, together with the skin, constitute the integumentary system. Alcoholic solutions are used for the treatment of onychomycosis due to their good absorption capacity through the nails.

Target

Identify each of the components and their association to evaluate possible side effects, as well as the role of the base (alcohol, glycerol, etc.) as excipient.

Basis

Since the faneras (organs of epithelial origin such as hair, feathers, claws, hooves) are difficult to penetrate by traditional excipients of ointments or liniments, the alcohol and the adjuvant contained in this preparation help the iodide solution to act as a fungicidal agent.

Formula:

1. Salicylic Acid (10% alcoholic solution)		5.0 mL
2. Iodide solution		10.0 mL
3. Cane alcohol	(c.b.p. to be completed)	10.0 mL

Material

1. Glass beaker (to measure the vehicle)
2. Two glass pipettes of 10 and 5 mL of glass
3. 100 mL glass beaker
4. Glass stirrer

Experimental part

1. In the glass put the alcohol, add the rest of the ingredients, mixing gently until homogenized.
2. The teacher will always be present for any problems or doubts that may arise.

Practice 12. Scratch Paste I

Introduction

In pharmacy, paste is a dosage form composed of powders and fats mixed in similar proportions. Vaseline is extremely versatile and is used worldwide to protect and repair dry skin, from dry, chapped hands to hard skin on heels, as well as for cosmetic purposes, such as softening lips or highlighting cheekbones. This means that it is often used to protect and repair the skin. Wearing your legs in the air causes the fairly common problem of chafing on the thighs. The friction of the skin added to the heat causes the area to become irritated and painful blisters are created that will prevent us from being able to walk with ease, between the thighs or crotch, inner thigh area near the groin, causing chafing on the skin. The use of vaseline as a vehicle for different drugs and active ingredients of medicinal plants is very old and the most economical, when it contains high proportions of finely dispersed solids in the excipient.

Target

Identify each of the components and their association to evaluate possible side effects, as well as the role of the base (petroleum jelly) as excipient.

Basis

Dermatological pastes are ointment-like mixtures containing starch (in this formulation it is corn starch), zinc oxide with astringent, antiseptic or protective properties, which is given a uniform pasty consistency with glycerin, vaseline or other fats. They usually have a higher proportion of pulverized substance than ointments; they are less greasy, but more absorbable than other preparations and should not contain sabulous particles (crystals or gritty).

Formula:

Corn or Rice Starch	25.0 g
2. Zinc Oxide	25.0 g
Glycerin	20.0 g
4. Solid petroleum jelly	20.0 g

Material

1. Granatary balance
2. Bain Marie
3. Metal spatula
4. 200 mL glass beaker

5. Lighter and tipié
6. Glass plate

Experimental part

1. In a glass plate, mix the Zinc Oxide and the starch with a little glycerin, adding each time a little more until a pasty and very smooth consistency, add this paste to the previously melted petroleum jelly (80 °C), and the rest of the glycerin, continue mixing until a smooth and homogeneous consistency.
2. Proceed to primary and secondary packaging and labeling of the product.
3. The teacher will always be present for any problems or doubts that may arise.

Practice 13. Scratch Paste II

Introduction

The use of petroleum jelly as a vehicle for different drugs and active ingredients of medicinal plants is very old and the most economical, when it contains high proportions of finely dispersed solids in the excipient.

Target

Identify each of the components and their association to evaluate possible side effects, as well as the role of the base (petroleum jelly) as excipient.

Basis

Dermatological pastes are ointment-like mixtures containing starch (in this formulation it is corn starch), zinc oxide with astringent, antiseptic or protective properties, which is given a uniform pasty consistency with glycerin, vaseline or other fats. They usually have a higher proportion of pulverized substance than ointments; they are less greasy, but more absorbable than other preparations and should not contain sabulous particles (crystals or gritty).

Formula:

Corn or Rice Starch	25.0 g
2. Zinc Oxide	25.0 g
Glycerin	20.0 g
4. Solid petroleum jelly	20.0 g
5. Lanolin	10.0 g

Material

1. Granatary balance
2. Bain Marie
3. Metal spatula
4. 200 mL glass beaker
5. Lighter and tipié
6. Glass plate

Experimental part

1. In a glass plate, mix the zinc oxide and starch with a little glycerin, adding a little more each time until a pasty and very smooth consistency is left, add this paste to the previously melted petroleum jelly and lanolin (80 °C), and the rest of the glycerin, continue mixing until a smooth and homogeneous consistency.

2. Proceed to primary and secondary packaging and labeling of the product.
3. The teacher will always be present for any problems or doubts that may arise.

Practice 14. Cosmetology. Facial Cream

Introduction

Cosmetology is the study and art of using cosmetics or products to beautify the physical appearance. It is the application of products to improve facial and body aesthetics using therapies for the skin, hair and nails. A cosmetic product is currently defined as any substance or preparation intended to be placed in contact with the various superficial parts of the human body (epidermis, hair and capillary system, nails, lips, and external genital organs) or with the teeth and oral mucous membranes, with the exclusive or main purpose of cleaning them, modifying their appearance and/or correcting body odors and/or protecting or maintaining them in good condition.

Target

To introduce the student to the field of cosmetology, in order to certify to the public that cosmetic products are guaranteed and supervised by pharmacists, which is why they are called "dermopharmaceuticals". Based on this idea, some cosmetic companies channel their products exclusively through the pharmacy office.

Basis

In the dermopharmaceutical and cosmetic market, there are very diverse formulations, from simple solutions (aqueous and oily), suspensions, gels and emulsions to solid forms such as pastes, bars, sticks, powders, creams, etc. Creams for the care of normal skin are intended to maintain optimal hydration of the stratum corneum.

They are usually non-ionic O/A emulsions suitably formulated. There are also specific A/O, in which the aqueous phase is present in a high percentage and which have moisturizing properties for the superficial layers of the skin, leaving a very porous lipid layer with a non-greasy appearance.

This formulation prepares an O/A emulsion duly formulated with specific moisturizing products (wetting agents) capable of maintaining or restoring the hydration of the upper layers of the epidermis and with a high percentage of fatty phase that helps against the dryness of our semi-desert environment.

Formula:

1. Stearic acid	20.0 g
Solid petroleum jelly	20.0 g
Liquid petroleum jelly	40.0 g

Glycerin 20.0 g

5. Triethanolamine 5.0 g

6. Distilled water c.b.p. desired consistency.

7. Aroma to taste

Material:

1. 400 mL glass beaker

Garnet balance

Metal spatula

Bain Marie

Experimental part:

1. Melt the solid petroleum jelly in a water bath (80 °C).
2. Once melted, remove it, add, always mixing constantly, the liquid petroleum jelly and the stearic acid previously melted at 60 °C followed by the glycerin and triethanolamine, adding them in the form of a fine thread without stopping mixing.
3. Add the water, always mixing until the desired semi-solid or semi-liquid consistency is obtained.
4. The teacher will always be present for any problems or doubts that may arise.

Practice 15. Cosmetology. Anti-wrinkle cream

Introduction

A cosmetic product is currently defined as any substance or preparation intended to be placed in contact with the various superficial parts of the human body (epidermis, hair and capillary system, nails, lips, and external genital organs) or with the teeth and oral mucosa, with the exclusive or main purpose of cleaning them, modifying their appearance and/or correcting body odors and/or protecting them or keeping them in good condition and recovering, as far as possible, a more youthful appearance, which is why these formulations are in continuous expansion.

Target

To introduce the student to the field of cosmetology, to guarantee to the public that cosmetic products are guaranteed and supervised by pharmacists, which is why they are called "dermopharmaceuticals". Based on this idea, some cosmetic companies channel their products exclusively through pharmacies.

Basis

In the dermopharmaceutical and cosmetic market, there are very diverse formulations, from simple solutions (aqueous and oily), suspensions, gels and emulsions to solid forms such as pastes, bars, *sticks,* powders, creams, etc. With creams for the care of normal skin, the aim is to maintain optimal hydration of the stratum and to develop an activity capable of blocking the metabolic mechanisms responsible for the appearance of the aesthetic alterations typical of senile skin.

They are usually non-ionic O/A emulsions suitably formulated. There are also specific A/O, in which the aqueous phase is present in a high percentage and which have moisturizing properties on the superficial layers of the skin, leaving a very porous lipid layer with a non-greasy appearance.

This formulation prepares an O/A emulsion properly formulated with specific moisturizing products (wetting agents) capable of maintaining or restoring the hydration of the upper layers of the epidermis and with a high percentage of fatty phase that helps against the dryness of our semi-desert environment.

The main ingredients also include anti-aging enzymes, antioxidant substances such as vitamin E and chelating systems.

Formula:

1. Beeswax	10.0 g
2. Lanolin	10.0 g
3. Olive Oil	75.0 g
4. Vitamin E	1 capsule

Material

1. Bain Marie
2. Granatary balance
3. Scalpel (to break the Vitamin E capsule)
4. Metal spatula

Experimental part

1. Melt the beeswax and lanolin together in a water bath (80 °C).
2. Remove to room temperature, adding the rest of the ingredients and mixing until a homogeneous and smooth consistency is obtained.
3. The teacher will always be present for any problems or doubts that may arise.

Practice 16. Cough Syrup

Introduction

Syrups (Arabic, sarab) are liquids of viscous consistency usually containing concentrated solutions of sugars, such as sucrose, in water or other liquid. Syrups have been used for a long time and before the discovery of sugar, they were prepared with honey. The liquids that usually make up syrups are distilled water, solutions, extractives, juices, and others. A syrup is a sweet substance that contains integrated medicines and is given especially to children for ingestion.

Their main purpose is to provide a remedy for a specific disease or group of diseases. The pleasant taste associated with them is an extra contribution that may depend on different elements, including sugar. They may contain alcohol as a way of contributing to their preservation. As for color, this may be variable or non-existent. Being syrups (potions) liquids for oral administration, they are usually dissolutions, emulsions or suspensions, containing one or more active ingredients in an appropriate vehicle.

Target

To introduce the student to the correct preparation of syrups, giving the correct concentration and bringing to boiling to form the invert sugar to increase the sweetening action. Based on the knowledge acquired in the theoretical part, the student will identify each one of the components and their association to evaluate the possible side effects, as well as the function of the syrup base as an antimicrobial protector.

Basis

Syrups are aqueous preparations with high sugar content, which gives them their characteristic consistency, the high proportion of sugar serves to hide the bad taste of the active ingredients and ensure their preservation. If there is an excessive amount of sugar, it crystallizes and water should be added to adjust the density, which should not be less than 1.32. If there is too little sucrose, there is a risk of proliferation of microorganisms.

Syrups should be stored in tightly covered bottles in cool places. Depending on their composition, authorized preservatives may sometimes be added at permitted concentrations.

Formula:

1. Sucrose	400.0 g
2. Distilled water	500.0 mL
3. Bee honey	300 g
4. Mullein alcohol extract	10.0 mL
5. Alcoholic extract of bougainvillea blossom flower.	10.0 mL
6. Alcoholic extract of Eucalyptus	10.0 mL
	2.0 mL
7. Guaiacol alcoholic solution (5%)	
8. Menthol (10% alcoholic solution)	10.0 mL
9. Camphor (5% alcoholic solution)	2.0 mL

Material

1. Granatary balance
2. 2 L beaker
3. Bunsen burner, with tipie or electric grill
4. 500 mL flask
5. Graduated glass pipettes, one for each solution
6. Large wooden spatula

Experimental part

Boil the water with the sucrose for 10 to 15 minutes (to form invert sugar), add the honey while hot, mix well with the spatula and add the alcoholic solutions one by one, mixing at each addition while the syrup is hot so that the alcohol evaporates.

3. The teacher will always be present for any problems or doubts that may arise.

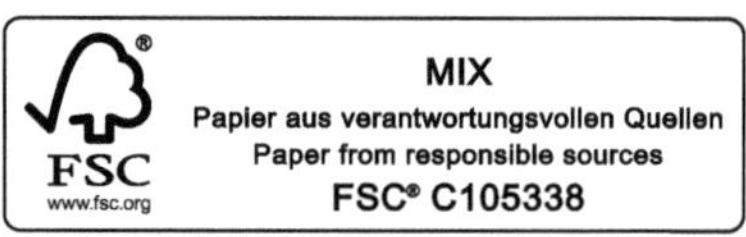

Printed by Books on Demand GmbH, Norderstedt / Germany